Feeling better

controlling pa[in and]
other sympto[ms]

This booklet is for you if you or [someone clos]e to you has cancer. It is a practical guide to drug and non-drug ways of dealing with pain and other symptoms caused by cancer.

If you are a patient your doctor or nurse may wish to go through the booklet with you and mark sections that are particularly important for you. You can make a note below of the main contacts and information that you may need quickly.

Specialist nurse/contact name	Family doctor
....	....
Hospital	**Surgery address**
Phone	*If you like you can also add:*
Treatments	**Your name** ....
....	**Address** ....
....	....

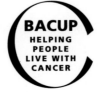

BACUP
HELPING
PEOPLE
LIVE WITH
CANCER

BACUP
HELPING
PEOPLE
LIVE WITH
CANCER

3 Bath Place, Rivington Street, London, EC2A 3JR

BACUP was founded by Dr Vicky Clement-Jones, following her own experiences with ovarian cancer, and offers information, counselling and support to cancer patients and their families.

We publish booklets on the main types of cancer, treatments, and ways of living with cancer. We also produce a magazine, *BACUP News,* three times a year.

Our success depends on feedback from users of the service. We thank everyone whose advice has made this booklet possible.

Administration 0171 696 9003
Cancer Information Service 0171 613 2121
Freeline (outside London) 0800 181199
Cancer Counselling Service 0171 696 9000 (London based)
BACUP Scotland 0141 553 1553

British Association of Cancer United Patients and their families and friends. A company limited by guarantee. Registered in England and Wales company number 2803321. Charity registration number 1019719. Registered office as above.

Medical consultant: Dr Maurice Slevin, MD, FRCP

Editor: Nikki Hill

Text: Jenny Bryan

Cover design by Alison Hooper Associates

Illustrations by Andrew Macdonald and Alexa Rutherford

Typeset and printed in Great Britain by Lithoflow Ltd., London

ISBN 1-870403-39-8

Contents

Introduction

This booklet has been written to help you understand more about some of the symptoms which may occur with cancer. Some are caused by the cancer itself, others are a result of treatment. You may experience one or more of these symptoms, or none at all. But they can all be controlled with help from you, your family and friends, and members of the medical and nursing team caring for you.

'Will I be in pain?' is a question commonly asked by people diagnosed with cancer. The answer is that one in three cancer patients have no pain at all. And a better understanding of the causes of pain, together with new, more effective ways of treating it, mean that there is rarely any need, at any stage, to suffer unmanageable pain. It is important to know that pain is not related to the extent of the cancer. Having pain does not necessarily mean that the cancer is advanced or more serious than if you had no pain.

Everyone feels pain differently and even people with the same disease have very different experiences. Pain is what you say hurts. And, like any other symptom of cancer, it should be treated according to your own particular needs.

In this booklet we describe the wide range of treatments available for controlling pain and other symptoms of cancer and we also look at some of the support services which can help you.

We can't advise you about the best treatment for yourself because this information can only come from your own doctor who is familiar with your medical history.

At the end of this booklet you will find a list of BACUP publications, some useful addresses and recommended books. If, after reading this booklet, you think it has helped you, do pass it on to any of your family and friends who might find it interesting. They too may want to be informed so that they can help you to cope with any problems that you may have.

Causes of pain

Pain may occur for a number of reasons. A cancer may press on the tissues around it or on a nerve. Infection can set up a painful reaction. People often forget that damage to tissues following surgery may be painful too.

Pain may also come from secondary tumours, called metastases. These are often a cause of bone pain. Sometimes, pain can occur in places well away from the original tumour. This is because nerves may carry pain between totally different parts of the body. So pain caused by a tumour in the chest may be felt in the shoulder or arm. Pain which arises in this way is called referred pain.

People with cancer should discuss any new pain with their doctor but it is important not to forget that you are just as prone to headaches, muscle pains and stomach aches as before your illness. It is understandable that someone with cancer tends to assume that a new ache or pain means that their illness is getting worse or the cancer has spread.

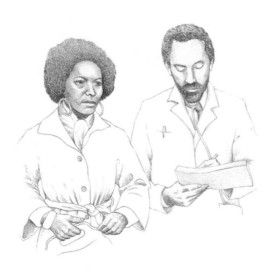

But often the pain has nothing to do with the cancer. Your doctor or nurse may well be able to put your mind at rest so it is always worth discussing any new pain with them.

Fear can make your pain worse, as can many other emotions including anxiety, depression and tiredness. This does not mean that cancer pain is 'all in the mind'. Symptoms of many physical illnesses, including asthma, heart disease and stomach ulcers are made worse by emotional upset. In all these conditions, as with pain from cancer, it is important to treat the emotional as well as the physical causes of the problem.

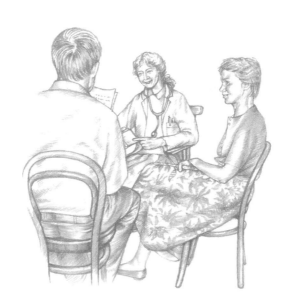

Describing pain

If you can describe your pain it will help the doctors and nurses work out the best way of treating it. The more you can tell them, the better the idea they can get about the possible cause. Here are some questions you might try to answer.

- Where is the pain? Is it in one part of your body or more? Or does it start in one place and gradually spread during the day?

- What is it like? Is it dull and aching, burning, or sharp and stabbing for example? Is it similar to any pain you have had before, like toothache or cramp? Is it near the surface or deep inside?

- How bad is it? Try to rate your pain by comparing it with pain you have experienced before, such as headache, back or period pain, sports injury, childbirth. If you were to rate your pain on a scale of one to ten, how would you rate it?

- Does anything make it better or worse? Do you feel better standing, sitting or lying down, for example? Does a hot-water bottle or ice-pack help? Or perhaps some pain-killers, such as aspirin? Can you distract yourself with a good book, music, TV etc?

- Is the pain there all the time? Does it come and go? Is it worse at night? Does it keep you awake? Does it wake you?

Don't feel you are being a nuisance or making a fuss. Go into as much detail as you can.

Medical treatments for pain

Common worries about pain control

Before looking at the drugs commonly used to control cancer pain, it is important to think about some of the worries you may have about starting on pain-killers.

Many people believe that they should put off using pain-killers for as long as possible - that they should only seek help when the pain is becoming unbearable. This is simply not true. There are plenty of effective pain-killers for all types of pain, so there is no need to 'save' them until your pain is severe. Taking pain-killers as soon as you are in pain will not make them less effective later on.

Sometimes a doctor will start by giving you a mild pain-killer and go on to prescribe a moderate or strong drug if and when it becomes necessary. Or, if you have severe pain, you may be given a strong pain-killer, such as morphine, straight away. This does not mean that the cancer is more serious, just that the pain is severe.

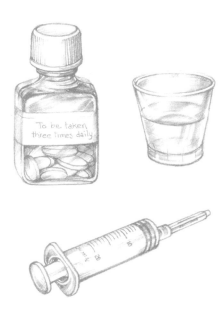

Do not be surprised if you are given other drugs such as anti-inflammatory agents, sleeping pills or antidepressants to take with your pain-killers. These will also help to control your pain, but in a different way from your pain-killers.

'Getting addicted' is another common worry. There is no danger of you becoming 'hooked' on drugs such as morphine, needing larger doses to satisfy your cravings like a drug addict. The dose you take will be carefully tailored to your own special needs and will only have to be increased if your pain gets worse. Many people stay on the same dose of morphine for many months. If your pain gets less the dose can easily be reduced under the supervision of your doctor.

When you are taking pain-killers always be sure to take your dose regularly. The aim is to prevent pain. So don't wait for your pain to come back before taking your drug or you will suffer unnecessarily while it is absorbed and starts to work.

Choosing a pain-killer depends on the type and severity of the pain being treated. Fortunately there is a very large range of pain-killing drugs available. In addition, there are other methods of relieving pain, such as radiotherapy. The aim therefore is to find the right combination of medical treatments to ensure the best possible pain control is achieved for each individual patient.

Any pain-killer dose should be enough to control pain right through until the next dose. If your pain tends to return before the next dose is due, be sure to tell your doctor or nurse so that a more effective dose or a different drug can be used. It takes time and care to get things exactly right. So do persevere and don't suffer in silence!

Mild drugs for pain relief

Aspirin and paracetamol are very effective pain-killers which can be bought from the chemist. Aspirin has the added advantage that it may reduce inflammation and swelling as well as relieving pain, but it can cause indigestion and stomach bleeding in some people. To reduce the risk of stomach problems it is always advisable to take the kind of aspirin which dissolves in water. Nor should aspirin normally be taken on an empty stomach or with alcohol. Paracetamol does not cause stomach problems.

Never use more aspirin or paracetamol than is recommended on the packet and be sure to tell your own doctor if you are already using one of these drugs so that any other treatment can be adapted accordingly. You can tell if any medicine or tablets you buy from the chemist contains either of these drugs as it should say so on the packet; check with the pharmacist if you are not sure.

You may well find that your doctor recommends you take either aspirin or paracetamol as well as other pain-killing drugs, such as those described in the next two sections. This is so that your pain can be tackled in more than one way. Aspirin, for example, works at where your pain is felt, while these other drugs work in the brain, where the pain is recorded.

Moderately powerful drugs for pain relief

Included in this group are drugs which contain codeine (Co-Dydramol, DF118), dextropropoxyphene (Distalgesic, Co-Proxamol), or buprenorphine (Temgesic). They work in the brain and nervous system and are available only on prescription from a doctor. They may cause drowsiness so you should find out how they affect you before attempting to do anything needing concentration, such as driving. These drugs are known to cause constipation, so it is advisable to ask your doctor to prescribe a laxative for you to take with these types of pain-killers. These drugs should not be taken with alcohol if you are going to do anything that requires concentration, such as driving.

Stronger drugs for pain relief

Morphine or diamorphine is the most commonly used of these drugs and can be taken in a variety of ways – as tablets, syrup, suppositories (inserted into the back passage), or by injection. As with any pain-killer it is important to find the most effective dose for each person. Two patients with the same type of cancer at the same stage of disease may require entirely different doses of morphine. It is usual to start at a low dose and build up gradually to get the best pain relief. The dose can be changed and/or other pain-killers used with the morphine so that the pain is kept under control.

Most cancer patients who are offered morphine ask if they will get addicted to the drug or become confused and unable to look after themselves. The answer is 'no'. As mentioned earlier, cancer patients, unlike drug addicts, do not need bigger and bigger doses of morphine to 'feed' a mental addiction. However, it is unwise to stop taking morphine suddenly. The dose of many drugs, including steroids and drugs to lower the blood pressure, should be reduced gradually and the same applies to morphine.

Like the pain-killers in the 'moderate' group morphine may cause drowsiness. This usually passes within a few days. People vary in how this affects them, but if you are planning to drive or to work with machinery you should test your general reactions and alertness. Do not, of course, drink alcohol if you are planning to drive or do anything that requires concentration. Take a friend out in the car on some quiet roads and see how you get on. Only if you are both confident that your concentration is not impaired should you consider driving regularly. It is also best to check with your GP first.

Morphine has two common side effects which can be relieved with other drugs. Constipation is so common that patients are advised to use a laxative throughout their treatment. Preferences vary between drugs which soften the stools and make them easier to pass and those which stimulate the bowel so that it pushes the stools along more quickly. A combination of the two types of product is often the best solution and your doctor will be able to advise you which ones to use.

Some people feel sick when they first start taking morphine so they are advised to use an anti-sickness drug (anti-emetic) at least for the first week of treatment. A dry mouth is an annoying, though less serious, side effect of drugs such as codeine and morphine. This does not require drug treatment and can be relieved by drinking plenty of liquid and sucking fresh pineapple slices.

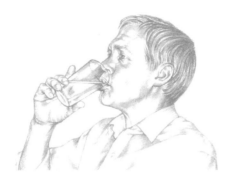

Take care about storing medicines which contain morphine. Make sure that they are properly labelled and lock them up or keep them out of reach of children. If you are worried about forgetting to take them, write a note to yourself and put it in a prominent place rather than leaving morphine on display or start a 'drug diary' to keep track of when your drugs are due to be taken.

Other helpful drugs

As an alternative to aspirin or paracetamol you may be prescribed a non-steroidal anti-inflammatory drug (NSAID). Like aspirin, these drugs work at where the pain is felt and they reduce inflammation and swelling too. They are especially good at treating pain caused by cancer involving the skin, muscle or bone. Since people vary in the way they respond to these drugs it is often worth trying a few different products to find the one which suits you best. Steroid drugs may be given alone or with other pain-killers when pain is caused by a tumour pressing on or damaging a nerve.

Steroids may increase the appetite and generally make people feel better. They have a few side-effects which are usually mild and disappear gradually once the treatment is over. These include weight gain, indigestion, high blood pressure and a slightly greater risk of getting infections.

It is impossible to overstress the importance of relieving anxiety and depression as part of the overall control of pain. Talking with family, friends or counsellors is very helpful. But you may also benefit from a short course of tranquillizers, such as diazepam. Diazepam is also used to relax muscles for those who have muscle spasm pain.

Antidepressants may also be helpful. They take about a week to work and are often given for several months. Sleeping pills, too, can be very useful for those who have trouble getting off to sleep, and can be used alongside pain-killers.

When pain is due to some underlying infection you are likely to be given antibiotic drugs, to treat the root of the problem.

Taking your drugs

If you are taking several different drugs you will probably find it helpful to draw up a chart listing the drugs, their doses and the time of day to take them. Your doctor or nurse can help you.

The aim is to make things as simple as possible. Wherever possible the doses of your drugs should be timed to coincide with one another. If one of the medicines has to be taken only once or twice a day, try to take it at the same time as one of the other drugs which has to be taken more often. By taking more than one medicine at a time you can cut down on the number of times each day when you have to remember to take your drugs.

For example, at breakfast you might be taking your morphine, a laxative and some aspirin. At lunch and dinner times, it may be just morphine and aspirin. And then, at night, half an hour before bed, you might be taking morphine, aspirin and a sleeping pill.

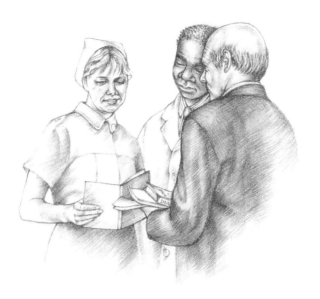

If you are worried about forgetting your drugs make sure there is room on your chart to tick off each dose. Or your nurse can probably provide you with a tray of containers for your medicines, labelled with the times at which to take them. Then at any time during the day, you can check that you are up to date.

You may also find it useful to keep a diary of how well your symptoms are being controlled. This will help the medical team too. They will be able to see whether the doses of any of your drugs need changing. Or, if you don't want to bother with a full diary, just make a note if your pain or other symptoms come back before your next dose of medicine is due.

Methods of giving drugs

Pain-killing drugs are usually taken by mouth (orally). There are oral forms of all the commonly used pain-killers. As we have already mentioned, some drugs, such as aspirin, are better taken in liquid form. And some people find it easier to swallow their drugs when they are dissolved in a drink. Alternatively, for those who have trouble swallowing, a number of pain-killing drugs are available as suppositories (which are inserted into the back passage).

Morphine is generally taken every four hours as a syrup, or mixed with a fruit drink as preferred. There is also a controlled release tablet. This is swallowed but the morphine comes out of the tablet very slowly, over a period of about twelve hours. Some people find this is more convenient than taking the drug every four hours. A controlled release suspension has also been developed which, like the tablets, releases morphine slowly over 12 hours. This is mixed in water and taken as a drink.

Morphine can also be given as an injection, but as easy-to-take oral forms have been developed fewer people have needed injections. Occasionally urgent treatment for severe uncontrolled pain is needed and injections can bring immediate relief because the drug gets straight into the bloodstream.

For patients whose pain is difficult to control with oral pain-killers, a continuous infusion of morphine into the body is often very effective. This method uses a syringe driver. A syringe of morphine is attached to a small pump and the drug is slowly pumped under the skin, or less commonly into a vein, through a needle. The rate at which the drug goes into the body can be adapted very carefully to the patient's changing needs. And, since the syringe driver is only the size of a cassette and clips easily onto your belt or into a specially designed small holster that fits under your arm, you can be up and around as usual.

Non-drug methods of pain control

Non-drug methods of pain control can be used alone or alongside pain-killing drugs. They include radiotherapy, transcutaneous electrical nerve stimulation (TENS), acupuncture, nerve blocks, hypnotherapy and relaxation techniques. Operations on the spinal cord, though rare, can be very helpful for pain that is not relieved by other methods.

Radiotherapy is a very effective way of controlling pain in the bones, especially the spine, thigh bones, pelvis and rib cage. It helps to relieve pain and enables the bone to build its strength again. The dose of radiotherapy used to treat pain is usually quite low and the treatment therefore has very few side effects other than slight tiredness. BACUP has a booklet on radiotherapy which we would be happy to send you.

The aim of **TENS** is to stimulate the nerves reaching the brain. This makes the body release its own natural pain-killers, the endorphins. TENS has been known to relieve cancer pain, especially if the pain is confined to specific parts of the body.

It is thought that acupuncture may work in a similar way to TENS and may be helpful for some cancer patients. A number of specialist NHS pain clinics offer these techniques and your GP or cancer specialist can refer you.

Nerve blocks can also be done at specialist pain clinics. The idea is to stop painful messages from getting to the brain by blocking the nerves themselves. This can be done with a long acting local anaesthetic, chemicals, freezing (cryotherapy) or heat (radiofrequency thermo-coagulation).

Hypnotherapy may be useful in helping to relieve cancer pain but is rarely effective on its own. However, self-hypnosis can be a valuable part of the whole relaxation process which is used to reduce the effect of emotional upset on pain. Your GP may have a list of local therapists who provide hypnotherapy or you can contact BACUP for further information.

Things your family can do for you

Many people assume that drugs are the only way to control cancer pain. In fact they are only one aspect of treatment. Sometimes, the simplest ways of making you feel more comfortable are overlooked. And there are a lot of things, on their own or together with medical treatment, that you and your family can do to make you feel better.

Are you sitting comfortably?

The way you sit or lie down can affect your pain, and what may feel comfortable at first may be painful 15 or 20 minutes later. Family or friends can help you change position as often as necessary. This will also reduce the risk of your skin becoming sore and inflamed as a result of sitting or lying still in one position for long periods. Sitting or lying on a sheepskin helps prevent this.

Rugs or bedding may need to be tidied or changed too. It is remarkable how much better people feel when they get back into a cool bed with fresh bed linen. V-shaped pillows or supports can help reduce back and neck ache and a bed cradle can keep the weight of blankets off aching limbs.

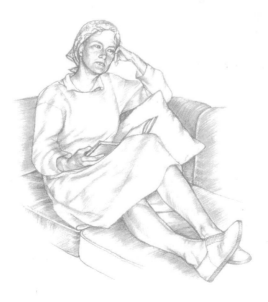

Feet may get forgotten. Foot rests and stools help relieve aches and pains and the special padded booties available, (like V-pillows, sheepskins and bed cradles, through your district nurse) serve the dual purpose of keeping feet warm and cushioned.

Hot or cold? Hot-water bottles and ice-packs can be effective pain relievers. Don't place them directly on bare skin but wrap them in a towel or piece of material. You may find that they only work for short periods at a time but don't give up on them, and alternate hot and cold.

Massage

You don't have to be an expert masseur to help relieve aching backs or limbs with gentle massage. By rubbing the painful area you will not only help to confuse the nerves sending pain messages to the brain, you will also help the muscles to relax. Why not try some refreshing herbal oils or lotions to moisturise the skin at the same time?

Diversional therapy

Watching TV, listening to music, or chatting to a friend won't make your pain go away, but it will help distract your attention, at least for a time. Sitting in a chair or lying in bed with nothing to do is depressing and even short periods of entertainment can help raise your spirits and enable you to cope better with your pain. Short, frequent visits from friends and relatives are probably better than longer ones. They are less tiring, help break up the day and are something to look forward to.

Getting things off your chest

We have already mentioned that anxiety and depression can make pain worse. People with cancer need to be able to talk about their worries and fears with those who are close to them. They may be anxious about their treatment or worried about coping at home. There may be real or imagined financial problems. Often, friends or relatives can help by getting more information from doctors and nurses or finding out about services which can help. Sometimes, there is little to say or do. Being there to listen and understand is enough.

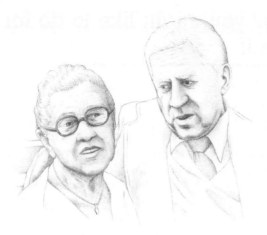

BACUP has booklets on talking about cancer which we can send you; *Who can ever understand?* is written for people with cancer and *Lost for words* is written for friends and relatives.

Spiritual help

Serious illness can force people to take life more seriously, to question the meaning of life and to stop taking things for granted. Some people who have religious beliefs may find their faith severely shaken by their cancer diagnosis. Even people who have never been regular worshippers may suffer spiritual as well as emotional pain. Questions like 'Is there life after death?' and 'Why should the people I love suffer?' are questions that some people find religious leaders, or others of a similar faith, can help them to answer.

Things you might like to do for yourself

You may find medication, visualisation, relaxation, or a combination of these techniques helpful in relieving your pain. Methods vary in detail but the overall aim is the same: to get rid of the stress and other emotional factors which may be making your pain worse. To learn these various techniques you can either go to classes or buy tapes, records or books. Your GP may well know of local relaxation classes, some of which are especially geared to the needs of cancer patients. BACUP has a booklet on complementary therapies which looks at some of these techniques. Here are some of the techniques commonly used.

Learning to relax and to get rid of the fears and anxieties – even if only for short periods each day – can play a useful part in your overall pain control, not least by reducing muscle tension. Relaxation involves getting to know particular groups of muscles around the body. Once you become aware that you can relax and contract stomach muscles, neck muscles and others individually or together you can start using the technique during stressful periods to reduce tension, and therefore pain.

Relaxation from within is encouraged by **autogenic training.** When you relax each part of your body – arms, legs, hands, feet, etc – you are encouraged to accompany this with thoughts of space, heaviness or warmth within those areas. Again, when you have mastered the basic techniques you can use them to assist with pain relief during difficult periods.

Visualisation helps you to bring happy relaxed pictures into your mind and use them to overcome some of your pain. By 'seeing' and 'hearing' images and sounds which bring you pleasure you can, to some extent, shut out symptoms of pain and discomfort.

Control of other cancer symptoms

People with cancer experience a wide range of symptoms –
some of them due to cancer, others caused by its treatment.
Often, these symptoms can be relieved by medical or non-
medical treatments or by a combination of both.

Eating problems

Many people lose their appetite and perhaps feel sick as well.
These may be symptoms of the illness itself or the result of
treatment, especially radiotherapy or chemotherapy. You may
be put off even by the sight and smell of food and your
worries about your illness may make things worse.

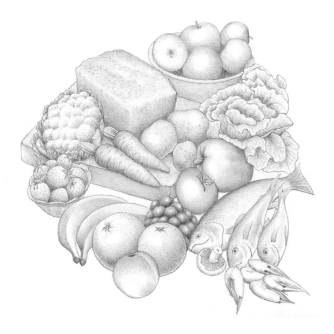

Small, frequent, simple meals are likely to be more tempting
than large plates of rich food. See BACUP's booklet *Diet and
the cancer patient* for hints and advice. This will also tell you
how to put more calories into your food without adding bulk
and will help you avoid losing weight since, once lost, it can
be difficult to regain. If you do start to lose weight, your

doctor may be able to prescribe a short course of steroid tablets to help you replace the lost weight.

Many cancer patients do gradually start to put their weight back on after their treatment has finished, but even so, weight loss can be distressing at the time. If this is so in your case, consider taking simple steps to improve your self-esteem, such as buying clothes a size smaller. BACUP's diet booklet has a section on how to cope with feelings about weight loss.

Try to get someone else to prepare food so that you do not feel too tired to eat by the time it is ready. During the most difficult times, try some of the high calorie drinks such as Complan and Build Up, and go back to solid foods when you feel better.

Feeling sick

If you feel sick or have trouble keeping food down, your doctor can prescribe an anti-emetic drug (anti-sickness drug) for you. These tablets should be taken regularly so that symptoms do not have a chance to come back. Unfortunately, it may not be possible to control entirely the sickness associated with some anti-cancer drugs but much can be done to reduce the symptoms. Sickness due to chemotherapy may last a few hours or at the most a few days. If it lasts longer, you should tell your doctor.

Sore mouth

Mouth ulcers can make your mouth so sore that you do not feel like eating. Some anti-cancer drugs, such as methotrexate and mitomycin C, are an occasional cause of mouth ulcers. Ideally, you should try to prevent the ulcers from forming by using mouthwashes at the first sign of soreness. You can buy these from your chemist; ask the pharmacist if you need help in choosing one. Your doctor may give you a mouthwash containing medicine to prevent ulcers, if he or she knows your drugs are likely to cause mouth ulcers.

Keeping your teeth clean may also help prevent infection setting in, but use a soft toothbrush to avoid aggravating painful gums.

For people who already have ulcers, an anaesthetic gel smeared onto the gums can help relieve the discomfort, as can cooling drinks and ice cubes. If your lips are also sore, try eating from a small spoon or drinking through a straw. Have a word with your doctor for advice about the best products for sore mouths.

If you are taking antibiotics you may sometimes develop a fungal infection, called thrush, in your mouth. This coats your tongue and can make eating unpleasant. Your doctor can prescribe medication to clear this infection.

Your bowels

Constipation and diarrhoea are the most common bowel problems people with cancer may get. When you are not feeling well it is easy to get out of your normal routine. You may not feel like eating and perhaps you are not getting your usual amount of exercise.

To prevent constipation, try to eat a balanced diet, including fibre-rich foods such as fresh fruit and vegetables, cereals and wholemeal bread, to keep your bowels moving. Drink plenty of fluids and try to get some exercise – even if it's only a short walk around the garden a couple of times a day.

If you do find yourself getting constipated, try sprinkling bran onto your cereal in the morning or your pudding in the evening. Eating prunes and figs and having hot lemon drinks are other useful constipation remedies you can do yourself. Tell your doctor if your constipation lasts for longer than three or four days, so that he or she can prescribe a laxative – either to soften the stools so that they can be passed more easily, or to stimulate your bowels into working normally.

If you are having diarrhoea, cut back on the foods rich in fibre and eat cooked fruit and vegetables instead of fresh ones. Keep away from fizzy drinks and spicy foods which encourage wind and stomach cramps. Avoid milk and dairy products such as cheese and yoghurt until the diarrhoea has stopped. It is also very important to replace the fluids your body is losing through the diarrhoea, so drink lots of liquids. If your diarrhoea persists for longer than 48 hours, you should tell your doctor. He or she can prescribe a drug which will help.

Breathing difficulties

Wheezing, shortness of breath and coughing may be problems for you. These symptoms may be related to the cancer, as in lung cancer, or caused by a chest infection or by a build-up of fluid on the surface of your lungs. Sometimes, fluid builds up inside the lungs themselves. Whatever the cause, however, breathing difficulties can be helped.

If you are wheezing or feeling short of breath because the tubes in your lungs have become too narrow, you can be given drugs to help the muscles around the tubes relax and to reduce any inflammation which may have caused the problem in the first place.

If there is a build-up of fluid on the surface of your lungs, the liquid can be carefully drawn out through a syringe, under a local anaesthetic. This can be done as often as is necessary, or a small tube can be stitched into your chest so that the liquid can be drained off continuously.

If an infection is causing you breathing difficulties this can be treated with antibiotics. Once the infection has cleared up, your breathing problems should improve.

You can buy cough mixtures from your chemist if coughing is a problem. Expectorants will loosen dry, chesty coughs and decongestants will relieve thick, mucus coughs. Your doctor should be able to advise you if you are not sure which you need.

Rapid breathing can be a very distressing symptom, but this too can be relieved. Morphine is very good at controlling breathing and bringing it down to a normal rate. If you are already on the drug for your pain control, the dose can be modified to cope with the breathing problems too.

If you have had radiotherapy to your chest, you may get a cough and feel mildly breathless for several weeks or months after your treatment has ended. This is due to inflammation in your lungs from the radiation and can be treated by a course of steroids. After taking the steroids for several weeks, your dose will gradually be reduced, and eventually stopped altogether, when the breathing problem has been relieved.

Remember, whatever your breathing problem, be sure to tell your doctor or nurse so that something can be done to help you.

Skin problems

Like breathing difficulties, skin problems such as itching or severe sweats may be due either to your cancer or to your treatment. If your skin is itchy, check that your clothes or bedding are not making it worse. Natural fibres such as wool and cotton are generally kinder to skin than artificial fibres. Be sure to avoid harsh washing powders, scented soaps and bubble baths and try unperfumed lotions and creams to soothe inflamed skin.

Night sweats are sometimes treated with steroids or non-steroidal anti-inflammatory drugs but, in general, light bed-clothes and a cool, well-aired room can do much to relieve the symptoms.

Pressure sores occur when areas of skin become inflamed and broken as a result of friction from clothing or bed-clothes. Thin, delicate skin over the joints such as the elbows, knees, hips, heels and at the base of the spine is especially prone to pressure sores. Once started, these sores are difficult to heal, particularly for people who are bed- or chair-bound and have poor circulation of their blood.

It is very important therefore to prevent pressure sores from developing in the first place. If you do need to spend a lot of time sitting down or lying in bed, make sure that you change your position at least every half an hour. Try sitting on an inflated cushion or lying on a soft sheepskin. Use pillows for support and keep the bed-clothes loose. A bed cradle under your sheet will keep the weight of the bed-clothes off your legs. All these aids are available free from your local nursing services.

Gently rub or massage areas of skin if they are beginning to get sore. Better still, get someone to do it for you! A massage is very relaxing as well as good for your skin. Unscented oils and lotions can also help to keep your skin soft and supple.

Always be on the look-out for patches of sore or inflamed skin, as these are early signs of pressure sores. Any such areas will need special attention, with frequent pressure relief and moisturising creams. If the skin does break down, the area must be kept very clean to try to prevent infection setting in. If the area does become infected, it must be cleaned frequently with antiseptic solutions and kept covered with a non-adhesive dressing. A course of antibiotics should help to clear the source of the infection.

Never keep quiet about early signs of pressure sores for fear of being thought a nuisance. The sores are quick to develop and will not go away by themselves. You will need help and advice from your district nurse to ensure that your skin heals properly and to prevent infection developing. Remember, once pressure sores are well-established they are difficult to get rid of.

The bladder

Bladder problems may occur if the cancer presses on or blocks the tubes from the bladder. The commonest reason for continence problems in men is an enlarged prostate which interrupts the normal flow of urine. Problems may also occur if there is damage to the nerves in the pelvis following surgery. Rarely, nerve damage may be due to a tumour pressing on the nerves in the spine. A bladder infection may cause you to pass urine more frequently and you may also have some pain on passing urine. These infections can be easily treated by antibiotics prescribed by your doctor.

Continence problems also arise because people who are chair- or bed-bound cannot get to a lavatory quickly enough. This is deeply distressing and embarrassing for previously active, independent people, but can be easily avoided by ensuring that assistance is always available or a commode easily to hand.

There is also a wide range of continence aids – pads, pants etc – for those with bladder control difficulties. This sort of protection has come a long way from the old-fashioned thick, bulging pads and creaking rubber pants. Instead, pads use materials which draw urine away from the body so that the wearer stays dry and comfortable. They are small and inconspicuous but secure enough to prevent embarrassing accidents.

For the bed-bound patient whose incontinence is more difficult to cope with or who is having trouble emptying his or her bladder a catheter can be inserted into the bladder so that urine is continuously drained away. Having a catheter used to be seen as a last resort. But it is simple, painless and greatly preferable to the infection, sores and discomfort which can accompany severe incontinence. Catheters only need to be changed about once a month and bottles and tubes can easily be concealed by bed-clothes or rugs.

Sleep disturbances

Most people with cancer have some trouble sleeping at some time during their illness. This may be linked with the emotional upset of their diagnosis and treatment or it may be due to disturbed sleep patterns. For example, if you feel tired and doze during the day you are likely to find it harder to sleep at night. Pain is another reason for disturbed sleep but this is effectively dealt with by good pain control.

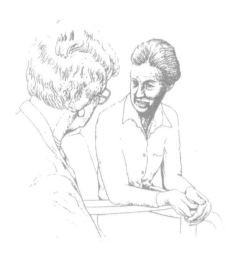

Relaxation, counselling and simply talking through the cause of any anxiety may be helpful for people whose insomnia is the result of emotional problems. Simple remedies such as a warm soothing bath, a milky drink, relaxing music and meditation may all help you to unwind before bed and put you in a more relaxed frame of mind for sleep. If problems persist, a short course of sleeping pills may help to re-establish a more normal sleeping pattern and get you over a particularly difficult patch.

When night-time insomnia is the result of frequent dozing during the day the answer may be to try to limit yourself to a single afternoon nap, of perhaps half an hour. Sort out a schedule for yourself during the day which involves regular walk-abouts, even if they are only round the garden or to the kitchen and back. Encourage friends and neighbours to drop in for a mid-morning coffee and chat and set yourself targets for doing things you enjoy, such as reading, arts and crafts. Your social services department or local volunteer organisation may be able to arrange transport to groups or for shopping etc.

It is very easy to slip into a routine of snoozing in front of the television all day and it may not be easy to push yourself into being more active. But if the alternative is hours spent tossing and turning at night it may be the only solution.

Fluid build up

Swollen ankles and legs

Some cancer patients become extremely worried if they notice their ankles and legs starting to swell. This can happen for several reasons; commonly it happens because you are not able to move about as much as usual. Although it may be frightening at the time, there is nothing to panic about if this symptom occurs. It can usually be easily controlled by diuretics (water tablets) which your doctor can prescribe.

Ascites

Certain types of cancer sometimes cause fluid (ascites) to build up in the abdomen so that it becomes swollen and uncomfortable. This can be relieved by inserting a small tube into the abdomen to drain the excess fluid. It usually needs to be done in hospital, with a local anaesthetic, and can be repeated as necessary. Sometimes this procedure can be done at home by your doctor. Alternatively, radiotherapy or chemotherapy may be able to prevent the ascites from coming back.

Lymphoedema

Fluid may also accumulate in tissues where the body's natural drainage system, the lymph glands, has been removed or damaged. This is especially common, for example, following mastectomy for breast cancer when the lymph glands under the arm are removed too. Fluid may build up in the arm on the affected side and this can be painful and embarrassing, especially if the swelling is severe. Massaging fluid away from the site of the build-up can help reduce the swelling, and elasticated sleeves can also keep the swelling down.

An elasticated sleeve attached to a pump - called a Flowtron - can be extremely effective in reducing the lymphoedema. Your nurse at the hospital or at home will be able to advise you on where to obtain a Flowtron and how to use it.

BACUP has a booklet on lymphoedema which we can send you.

Anxiety and depression

Anxiety and depression are two of the commonest emotional symptoms of cancer. It is natural to feel anxious and depressed, especially when you first hear your diagnosis, or during treatment. Questions like 'How will I cope?', 'What is going to happen?', 'Will I get better?', and 'Will the treatment work?' will probably flash through your mind.

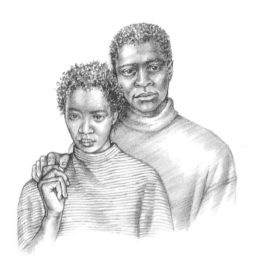

Sometimes anxiety may be expressed as physical symptoms such as a dry mouth, muscle pains, rapid heartbeats or indigestion. Feeling depressed can make it difficult to get to sleep and to concentrate, and can make you feel very tired and lethargic.

Voicing your fears will help others to help you. Practical help at home, financial advice if you cannot work, someone to listen while you talk, will all help to relieve your anxieties and lift your depression. Some GPs run counselling sessions to give you more time to talk over your worries, or they can put you in touch with trained counsellors or psychotherapists. BACUP offers counselling at its London and Glasgow offices. The Counselling Service can give you further information about counselling services in your area.

Sometimes anxiety and depression do need medical treatment. The physical symptoms they produce may occur days or weeks after diagnosis, but if they persist for more than three or four weeks, medical treatment may be necessary to relieve them.

Both anxiety and depression can be treated by psychological therapy, in which you learn ways of coping better with cancer-related stress. Occasionally, a course of antidepressant drugs for depression or a short course of tranquillizers for severe anxiety are helpful and these can be prescribed by your doctor.

Sources of help

Pain and symptom control form a very important part of the care of cancer patients and hundreds of doctors and nurses throughout the country specialise in this aspect of treatment. They are based in hospitals, hospices, continuing care units and pain clinics. There are also many home care teams of doctors and nurses who will visit you in your home and ensure that your symptoms are well controlled.

When you are at home your GP will be responsible for your day-to-day care. He or she can ask local district nurses to visit you when necessary. Your GP should also be aware of the more specialist pain and symptom control services in your area and can arrange for you to see them. You can ask to be referred to them.

What is available will depend on where you live. But whatever the system in your area, the most important thing is that you, your family, your GP and the specialist services know who is supervising your pain control. Day and night you should be able to get immediate help and advice, by telephone or in person.

Macmillan nurses: The main specialist continuing care service for cancer patients comes in the form of the fourteen Macmillan units and some 600 nurses provided by the Cancer Relief Macmillan Fund.

They operate from district general hospitals or through your local community nursing services. Macmillan units are set up by the Cancer Relief Macmillan Fund and the running costs are paid for by the local district health authority. These units are staffed by doctors and nurses specially trained in all the techniques for pain and symptom control. They offer in-patient care when required but otherwise aim to help people live as normally as possible at home.

Marie Curie nurses provide day or night care of cancer patients in their own homes. Whereas the Macmillan nurse tends to call in and advise specifically on symptom control, Marie Curie nurses can stay for longer periods and provide more general nursing care. They will also stay overnight if necessary so that the main carer can get a break. The local community nursing service will be able to provide details. In addition, Marie Curie Cancer Care runs eleven homes for cancer patients for long or short stay care.

Hospices also specialise in the continuing care of cancer patients. The Hospice Information Service has a directory of hospice services throughout the country. Some of these offer in-patient care only but many also run home care teams. Often, cancer patients spend a few days or weeks in a hospice having their symptoms sorted out and then return home to the care of their GP and community-based nurses with the help, support and advice of the hospice home care team. Your GP will know of the hospice services available in your area.

Hospices will help any patient with cancer who needs advice about controlling pain or any other symptoms. They do not only deal with dying or very seriously ill patients.

Alternatively, cancer patients who cannot look after themselves at home and have no regular carers may spend longer periods in a hospice.

Hospital support care teams specialise in symptom control for cancer patients in hospital and in the community. Referrals are generally made though the consultant in charge of the case, your GP or district nurse. You may also refer yourself. Nurses in these teams liaise closely with nursing services in a patient's local district so that when he or she goes home, help is still available for symptom control. A few specialised hospitals have palliative care units to sort out problems which patients are having trouble dealing with at home.

Pain clinics specialise in the treatment of all types of chronic pain, not just pain due to cancer. They are generally part of the district general hospital and are under the supervision of one or more consultant anaesthetists. The doctors and nurses who work in pain clinics are skilled in the use of all the drug and non-drug methods of pain control discussed in this booklet but specialise, in particular, in the use of nerve blocks. Patients are usually seen as outpatients to sort out specific pain problems which might be relieved by nerve blocks, acupuncture or TENS and their day-to-day care is then managed by their GP.

Sick pay and benefits

Incapacity Benefit has replaced Invalidity Benefit and Sickness Benefit. There are three rates of Incapacity Benefit: a short-term lower rate, a short-term higher rate, and a long-term rate.

If you are employed and unable to work, you employer will pay you Incapacity Benefit at the lower short-term rate for the first twenty-eight weeks. If, after this period, you are still unable to work you can claim the short-term higher rate of benefit from the Benefits Agency. After one year, if you are still unable to work, you can claim long-term Incapacity Benefit.

People who are unemployed will need to transfer from Unemployment Benefit to the short-term lower rate of Incapacity Benefit. This short-term lower rate of Incapacity Benefit is also available for up to one year after reaching state pension age.

If you are ill and not at work, do remember to ask your family doctor for a medical certificate to cover the period of your illness. If you are in hospital, ask the doctor or nurse for a certificate, which you will need to claim benefit. You may also be required to take a medical test to assess whether or not you are eligible for benefit.

The Benefits Agency have a form (IB201) which outlines all these benefits and others to which you may be entitled. You can get a copy by ringing 0800 868 868. Your local Citizens' Advice Bureau and Social Services office will also be able to advise you about the benefits to which you are entitled. Their addresses and telephone numbers are in the 'phone book.

BACUP's services

Cancer Information Service

This service is staffed by specially trained cancer nurses. If you ring or write to us, your phone call or letter will always be answered by a nurse who can give you information on all aspects of cancer and its treatment and who will offer practical and emotional support, whether you have cancer yourself or are the friend or relative of someone with cancer. A computerised directory and a library of resources are used by the nurses to provide information to anyone who enquires about treatment, research, support groups, therapists, counsellors, financial assistance, insurance, home nursing services and much more. The nurse can also send you any of our other booklets which might be helpful.

The Cancer Information Service is open to telephone enquiries from 10 am to 7 pm, Monday to Thursday, and until 5.30 pm on Friday. The number is 0171 613 2121 if you are ringing from London. You can call the service free of charge from outside the 0171 and 0181 telephone districts on 0800 18 11 99.

Cancer Counselling Service

Emotional difficulties linked to cancer are not always easy to talk about and are often hardest to share with those to whom you are closest. Skilled counsellors help people to talk about their thoughts, feelings and ideas and perhaps untangle some of the difficulties and confusion that living with cancer brings.

BACUP offers a face-to-face and group counselling service based at its London offices. A face-to-face counselling service is also available at BACUP Scotland in Glasgow. We can give you information about counselling services in your area, and discuss with you whether counselling would be helpful for you. For more information or to make an appointment with BACUP's Counselling Service, please ring 0171 696 9000 (London) or 0141 553 1553 (Glasgow) between 10 am and 5 pm, Monday to Friday.

Useful organisations

BACUP
3 Bath Place
Rivington Street,
London
EC2A 3JR
Office: 0171 696 9003

BACUP Scotland
(Cancer Counselling Service)
30 Bell Street
Glasow
G1 1LG
Office: 0141 553 1553

Cancer Information Service
Freephone (outside London): 0800 18 11 99
Inside London: 0171 613 2121
Open Monday-Thursday 10am-7pm, Friday 10am-5.30pm

Cancer Counselling Service
London: 0171 696 9000
Glasgow: 0141 553 1553

Jersey BACUP
6 Royal Crescent, St Helier, Jersey JE2.
Tel: 01534 89904 Freephone: 1200 275
In addition to providing a link with BACUP's Cancer Information Service in the Channel Islands, Jersey BACUP runs a local cancer support group and trained local volunteers give support over the telephone, and in the local hospital.

Hospice Information Service
St Christopher's Hospice, Lawrie Park Road, Sydenham,
London SE26 6DZ
Tel: 0181 778 1240/9252
Provides information and a directory of all hospice services – in-patient, home care and day care – in the UK and Ireland.

Sue Ryder Foundation
Cavendish, Sudbury, Suffolk CO10 8AY
Tel: 01787 280 252
Runs six homes for the continuing care of people with cancer.

Disabled Living Foundation
380-384 Harrow Road, London W9 3HU
Tel: 0181 289 6111
*Has information on equipment and aids for people with all
disabilities including those caused by cancer eg: incontinence
aids.*

CancerLink

17 Britannia Street
London WC1X 9JN
Tel: 0171 833 2451

9 Castle Terrace
Edinburgh EH1 2DP
Tel: 0131 228 5557

*Offers support and information on all aspects of cancer in
response to telephone and letter enquiries. Acts as a resource
to over 450 cancer support and self-help groups throughout
the UK, and publishes a range of publications on issues about
cancer.*

Cancer Care Society (CARE)
21 Zetland Road, Redland, Bristol BS6 7AH
Tel: 01179 427419 or 01179 232302

*Offers emotional support and practical help where possible
through support groups around the country. Telephone and
one-to-one counselling, telephone link service, holiday
accommodation.*

Cancer Relief Macmillan Fund
15-19 Britten Street, London SW3 3TZ
Tel: 0171 351 7811

*Provides home care nurses through the Macmillan Service and
financial grants for people with cancer and their families.*

Marie Curie Cancer Care
28 Belgrave Square, London SW1X 8QG
Tel: 0171 235 3325

*Runs eleven centres (hospices) throughout the UK, and a
community nursing service which supplements the District
Nursing Service and supports cancer patients and their carers
in conjunction with Health Authorities.*

Tak Tent Cancer Support – Scotland
The Western Infirmary, Block 20, Western Court,
100 University Place, Glasgow G12 6SQ
Tel: 0141 211 1932 (helpline)

Provides information, support and counselling for cancer patients, their relatives and professional staff involved in their care. Network of support groups throughout Scotland.

Tenovus Cancer Information Centre
College Buildings, Courtenay Road, Splott, Cardiff CF1 1SA
Tel: 01222 497700
　　 0800 526527 (Freephone helpline)

Provides an information service on all aspects of cancer. Operates a drop-in centre, helpline and support groups.

The Ulster Cancer Foundation
40-42 EglantineˈAvenue, Belfast BT9 6DX
Tel: 01232 663439 (helpline)
　　 01232 663281 (admin)

Provides a cancer information helpline, information and resource centre.

Recommended reading list

Robert Twycross
Oral Morphine: Information for Patients, Families & Friends
Beaconsfield
(ISBN 0-906584-12-4)

Rachel Clyne
Cancer: Your Life, Your Choice
Wellingborough, Thorsons Publishing Group
(ISBN 0-7225-21-030)

H. Smedley, K. Sikora and R. Stepney
Cancer: What it is and how it is treated
Oxford, Basil Blackwell
(ISBN 0-631-14041-7)

Chris and Sue Williams
Cancer: A guide for patients and their families
Chichester, Wiley
(ISBN 0-471-91017-1)

Jenny Bryan and Joanna Lyall
Living With Cancer
Penguin
(ISBN 0-14-009409-1)

Carolyn Faulder
A Special Gift: The Story of Dr Vicky Clement-Jones and the Foundation of BACUP
London, Michael Joseph
(ISBN 0-7181-3442-7)

Nira Kfir and Maurice Sleven
Challenging Cancer: From Chaos to Control
London, Tavistock/Routledge
(ISBN 0-415-06344-2)

Publications available from BACUP

Understanding:

Acute lymphoblastic leukaemia
Acute myeloblastic leukaemia
Cancer of the bladder
Primary bone cancer
Brain tumours
Cancer of the breast
Cervical smears
Cancer of the cervix
Chronic lymphocytic leukaemia
Chronic myeloid leukaemia
Cancer of the colon and rectum
Hodgkin's disease
Kaposi's sarcoma
Cancer of the kidney
Cancer of the larynx
Cancer of the liver
Cancer of the lung

Lymphoedema
Malignant melanoma
Cancer of the mouth and throat
Myeloma
Non-hodgkin's lymphoma
Cancer of the oesophagus
Cancer of the ovary
Cancer of the pancreas
Cancer of the prostate
Cancer of the skin
Cancer of the stomach
Soft tissue sarcomas
Cancer of the testes
Cancer of the thyroid
Cancer of the uterus
Cancer of the vulva

Living with cancer series:

Understanding chemotherapy
Understanding radiotherapy
Feeling better: controlling pain
   and other symptoms of
   cancer
Coping with hair loss
Diet and the cancer patient
Understanding bone marrow and
   stem cell transplants
Tamoxifen factsheet
Complementary therapies
   and cancer

Coping at home:
   caring for someone with
   advanced cancer
Understanding secondary
   breast cancer
Facing the challenge of
   advanced cancer
Lost for words:
   how to talk to someone
   with cancer
Who can ever understand?
   – talking about your cancer
Sexuality and cancer